HOW TO HAVE THE 100% INTELLIGENT QUOTIENT

SIMPLE SECRETS TO AN AMAZING AND PERFECTLY WORKING IQ

KARYN SAWYERR (PhD)

Copyright©2021 KARYN SAWYERR

All rights Reserved

TABLE OF CONTENTS

INTRODUCTION

CHAPTER ONE

WHAT IS INTELLIGENT QUOTIENT?

CHAPTER TWO

FACTORS INFLUENCING INTELLIGENT QUOTIENT
DETERMINANT OF INTELLIGENT QUOTIENT
FACTORS THAT CONTRIBUTE POSITIVELY TO YOUR INTELLIGENT QUOTIENT
FACTORS THAT CONTRIBUTE NEGATIVELY TO YOUR INTELLIGENT QUOTIENT
OTHER NEGATIVE LIFESTYLE CHOICES AND THE IMPLICATIONS

CHAPTER THREE

WAYS AT WHICH YOU CAN IMPROVE YOUR INTELLIGENT QUOTIENT
OTHER BASIC APPROACHES TO IMPROVE YOUR LEVEL OF INTELLIGENCE

CHAPTER FOUR

THE SIGNIFICANCE OF MENTAL WELLNESS

CHAPTER FIVE

THE CONNECTION AMONG DEPRESSION AND COGNITIVE DECLINE

WHAT EXPERTS ARE SAYING

IS THERE AN ASSOCIATION AMONG DESPONDENCY AND COGNITIVE DECLINE?

HOW DOES DEPRESSION CAUSE COGNITIVE DECLINE?

DIFFERENT REASONS FOR COGNITIVE DECLINE
IS COGNITIVE DECLINE AND SADNESS TREATABLE?
TREATING THE REASON
ADAPTING TO COGNITIVE DECLINE
WHAT CAN BE DONE TO PROTECT COGNITION?

CHAPTER SIX

THE PLACE OF NUTRITION

CHAPTER SEVEN

THE PLACE OF EXTRACURRICULAR-EXERCICES, GAMES

CHAPTER EIGHT

CONCLUSION

INTRODUCTION

Very much like we deal with all aspects of our body, our mind likewise requires such consideration and treatment.

Taking a closer look at the design of the brain through scans will empower us to see the value in its sensitivity and the delicate nature, we may have to look for the directions and counsel from neuroscientist or neurosurgeons to empower us see the value in the significance of the mind.

You cannot practically do anything with an inactive brain, when it stops, pretty much every movement including the body inside or remotely stops.

Besides that, we do not only need our mind to be dynamic yet additionally to help reason typically, tackle fundamental issues, and adapt to difficulties identifying with our reality and others.

Instructions to do every one of these and manage difficulties will rely entirely upon our degree of the intelligent quotient

CHAPTER ONE

WHAT IS INTELLIGENT QUOTIENT?

Knowledge is characterized as the overall mental critical thinking abilities of a person. It is the psychological capacity associated with adapting rapidly, analogies, ascertaining, thinking, seeing connections, and so forth.

Above all else, let me clarify what I mean when I give the signal "Intelligent quotient". Honestly, I'm not simply looking at expanding the volume of realities or pieces of information you can amass, or what is alluded to as solidified knowledge—this is not familiarity or retention preparing—it's practically the inverse, really. I'm looking at expanding your liquid insight, or your ability to learn new data, hold it, at that point utilize the new information as an establishment to tackle the following issue, or become familiar with the following new expertise, etc.

Presently, while working memory is not inseparable from knowledge, working memory corresponds with insight generally. To create an effectively shrewd yield, a decent working memory is really significant. So to benefit as much as possible from your insight, improving your functioning memory will help this essentially—like utilizing the absolute best and most recent extra parts to assist a machine with playing out its pinnacle.

This brings home focuses from this exploration this examination is pertinent because they found that:

1. Liquid intelligent is teachable.

2. The preparation and resulting gains is portion subordinate—which means, the more you train, the more you acquire.

3. Anybody can expand their psychological capacity, regardless of what their beginning stage is.

4. The impact can be acquired via preparing on undertakings that do not take after the test questions.

So—considering the entirety of this, I have thought of five essential components engaged with expanding your liquid insight, or psychological capacity. As I said, it is illogical to continually rehearse the double n-back errand or varieties thereof consistently for the remainder of your life to receive intellectual rewards. However, it is not unrealistic to receive the way of life changes that will have something very similar—and surprisingly more prominent psychological advantages. These can be carried out each day, to get you the advantages of extreme whole mental preparing, and should move to gains in generally speaking and intellectual working also.

These five essential standards are:

1. Look for Curiosity

2. Challenge Yourself

3. Think Inventively

4. Do Things The most difficult way possible

5. Organization

Any of these things without anyone else is extraordinary, yet if you truly need to work at your outright intellectual best, you ought to do every one of the five, and as regularly as could be expected. Truth be told, I carry on with my life by these five standards. On the off chance that you embrace these as major rules, I promise you will perform at your pinnacle capacity, outperforming even what you trust you can do—all without counterfeit improvement. The most awesome thing: Science do upholds are these standards via information!

1. Look for Curiosity

It is no accident that genius like Einstein was gifted in different zones, or polymaths, as we like to allude to them. Genius are continually searching out novel exercises, learning another space. It's their character.

There is just a single attribute out of the "Enormous Five" from the Five-Factor Model of character (Abbreviation: Sea, or Transparency, Reliability, Extroversion, Suitability, and Neuroticism) that connects with the level of intelligence and the quality of Receptiveness to new experience. Individuals who rate high on

Receptiveness are continually looking for new data, new exercises to participate in, new things to learn—new encounters when all is said and done

At the point when you look for curiosity, a few things are going on. Most importantly, you are making new synaptic associations with each new movement you take part in. These associations expand on one another, expanding your neural action, making more associations with expanding on different associations—learning is occurring.

A space of interest in late exploration in neural pliancy as a factor in singular contrasts is insight. Versatility is alluding to the number of associations made between neurons, how that influences resulting associations, and how durable those associations are. Fundamentally, implies how much new data you can take in and on the off chance that you can hold it, rolling out enduring improvements to your brain. Continually presenting yourself to new things helps place your brain in a prepared state for learning.

Curiosity additionally triggers dopamine which gets the inspiration going, yet it animates neurogenesis—the formation of new neurons—

and readies your mind for learning. You should simply take care of the yearning.

Magnificent learning condition = Novel Movement—>triggers dopamine—>creates a higher inspirational state—>which fills commitment and primes neurons—>neuro-beginning can happen + expansion in synaptic versatility (expansion in new neural associations or learning).

As a development of the Jaeggi study, specialists in Sweden tracked down that following 14 hours of preparing working memory for more than 5 weeks, there was an increase of dopamine D1 restricting potential in the prefrontal and parietal spaces of the mind. This specific dopamine receptor, the D1 type, is related to neural development and improvement, in addition to other things. This increment in versatility, permitting more prominent restricting of this receptor, is something excellent for augmenting intellectual working.

To drive home the point: Be an "Einstein". Continuously look to new exercises to draw in your psyche—extend your psychological skylines. Become familiar with an instrument. Take a craftsmanship class. Go to an exhibition hall. Find out about another space of science. Be an information addict.

2. Challenge Yourself

There are totally heaps of horrendous things composed and elevated on the most proficient method to "train your mind" to "get more astute". At the point when I discuss "mind preparing games", I'm alluding to the remembrance and familiarity type games, proposed to speed up handling, and so on, like Sudoku, that they advise you to do in your "leisure time" (total ironic expression, in regards to expanding insight). I will break a portion of that stuff you've recently found out about mind preparing games. Here goes: They do not work. Singular brain preparing games do not make you more brilliant—they make you more capable at mind preparing games.

Presently, they do fill a need, yet it is fleeting. The way to getting something out of those kinds of psychological exercises kind of identifies with the primary guideline of looking for curiosity. When you are involved in one of those psychological exercises in the mind preparing game, you need to proceed onward to the following testing action.

Sort out some way to play Sudoku, Fantastic! Presently move along to the following kind of testing game.

A couple of years prior, science needed to check whether you could expand your psychological capacity by strongly preparing novel mental exercises for a time of a little while. They utilized the computer game Tetris as the novel action and utilized individuals who had never played the game as subjects.

What they found, was that after preparing for half a month on the game Tetris, the subjects encountered an increase in cortical thickness, just as an expansion in cortical action, as confirmed by the increase in how much glucose was utilized in that space of the brain. Fundamentally, the brain utilized more energy during those preparation times and built up in thickness—which implies more neural associations, or recently scholarly aptitude—after this extraordinary preparation. Listen to this: After that underlying blast of intellectual development, they saw a decrease in both cortical thicknesses, just as the measure of glucose utilized during that task. Be that as it may, they stayed similarly as great at Tetris; their ability did not diminish. The mind examines showed less brain movement during the game-playing event, rather than improving, as in the earlier days. Why the drop? Their brains got more proficient. When their brain sorted out some way to play Tetris and be great at it, it got languid. It did not have to function as difficult to play the game well, so the intellectual energy and the glucose headed off to someplace else all things considered.

Effectiveness is not your companion with regards to psychological development. To keep your brain making new associations and keeping them dynamic, you need to continue proceeding onward to another difficult action when you arrive at the place of dominance in the one you are participating in. You need to be in a consistent condition of slight distress, attempting to scarcely accomplish whatever it is you are attempting to do, as Einstein insinuated in his statement. This causes your brain to remain alert, in a manner of speaking.

3. Think Innovatively

At the point when I say thinking innovatively will assist you with accomplishing neural development, I'm not looking at painting an image, or accomplishing something refined, as we talked about in the main standard, Looking for Curiosity. At the point when I discuss imaginative reasoning, I'm discussing inventive discernment itself, and what that implies the extent that the cycle going on in your brain.

As opposed to prevalent thinking, innovative reasoning does not rise to "thinking with the correct side of your brain". It includes enlistment from the two parts of your brain, not the perfect. Innovative insight includes unique reasoning (a wide scope of points/subjects), making a distant relationship between thoughts, exchanging to and fro among traditional and unusual reasoning (psychological adaptability), and producing unique, original thoughts that are likewise suitable to the movement you are doing. To do this well, you need both the right and left sides of the equator working related to one another.

Researcher opening the Speed (Brain science of Capacities, Skills, and Mastery) Center has been on a journey to comprehend the basic idea of knowledge, yet additionally to discover manners by which anyone individual can boost their insight through preparing, and particularly, through instructing in schools.

Recommendations

"The fundamental thought of the middle is that capacities are not fixed but instead adaptable, that they're modifiable, and that anybody can change their capacities into capabilities, and their skills into aptitude," "We're particularly intrigued by how we can assist individuals with adjusting their capacities so they can be better ready to confront the errands and circumstances they will go up against throughout everyday life."

They needed to see whether by instructing students to think imaginatively (and basically) about an issue, also concerning memory, they could get them to

(i) Learn more about the subject,

(ii) Have more fun learning

(iii) Transfer that information acquired to different spaces of scholastic execution. They likewise needed to check whether by fluctuating the educating and appraisal strategies, they could forestall "instructing to the test" and get the student to really learn more as a rule.

Basically overall, the understudies in the experimental group, the ones encouraged to utilize innovative strategies got higher last grades in the school course than the benchmark group educated with customary techniques and evaluations. In any case, just to make things reasonable—he likewise gave the experimental group the same logical sort test that the standard students got (a different decision test), and they scored higher on that test also. That implies they had the option to move the information they acquired utilizing inventive, multimodal showing strategies, and score higher on a totally extraordinary intellectual trial of accomplishment on that equivalent material. Sound recognizable.

4. Do Things the most difficult way possible

I referenced before that effectiveness is not your companion if you are attempting to expand your insight. Sadly, numerous things in life are fixated on attempting to make everything more productive. This is so that we can accomplish more things, in a more limited measure of time, an exhausting minimal measure of physical and mental energy conceivable. In any case, this is not helping your mind.

Take one object of current accommodation, GPS. GPS is an astounding development. I'm one of those individuals GPS was concocted for. My ability to know east from west is horrible. I get lost constantly. So when GPS went along, I was sending up a little prayer of thanks. Be that as it may, guess what? After utilizing GPS for a brief timeframe, I found that my internal compass was more terrible. On the off chance that I neglected to have it with me, I was significantly more lost than previously. So when I moved to Boston—the city that blood and gore flick and bad dreams about getting lost are designed according to—I quit utilizing GPS.

I would not lie—it was agonizing as hellfire. I had a new position that elaborate voyaging everywhere on the little hiding spots of Boston, and I got lost every day for in any event a month. I got lost so much; I thought I planned to lose my employment because of persistent delay (I even got queried for it). However, on schedule, I began learning my way around, because of the sheer measure of training I was getting at route utilizing only my brain and a guide. I started to really get a feeling of where things in Boston were, utilizing rationale and memory, not GPS. I can in any case recollect how glad I was the day a companion was visiting the area and I had the option to successfully discover his lodging downtown with just a name and an area portrayal to go on—not so much as a location. It resembled I had moved on from navigational mindfulness school.

Innovation does a great deal to make things in life simpler, quicker, more proficient, however here and there our psychological abilities can endure because of these alternate ways and hurt us over the long haul. Presently, before everybody begins shouting and messaging my trans-humanist companions to say that I've trespassed by destroying tech—that is not what I'm doing.

Take a closer look at it thusly: Heading to work takes less actual energy, saves time, and it's presumably more helpful and charming than strolling. Not a serious deal. In any case, on the off chance that you drove wherever you went, or consumed your time on earth on a Segway, even to go extremely brief distances, you would not use any actual energy. Over the long haul, your muscles will decay, your actual state will debilitate, and you'll most likely put on weight. Your general wellbeing will most likely decrease subsequently.

Your brain needs practice too. If you quit utilizing your critical thinking abilities, your spatial abilities, your intellectual abilities, your intellectual abilities—how would you anticipate that your brain should remain fit as a fiddle—never mind improve? Consider current comforts that are useful, however, when dependent on something over the top, can hurt your expertise in that space. Interpretation programming: stunning, however, my multilingual abilities have declined since I began utilizing it more. I've presently constrained myself to battle through interpretations before I look into the right arrangement. The equivalent goes for spell-checking and autocorrect. Truth be told, I think autocorrect was one of the most exceedingly awful things at any point created for the headway of cognizance. You realize the PC will get your slip-ups, so you plug along, not in any event, considering how to spell any longer. Because of long stretches of depending on autocorrect and spell-check, as a country, would we say we are more terrible spellers? (I would cherish somebody to examine this.)

There are times when utilizing innovation is justified and fundamental. However, there are times when it's smarter to deny alternate ways and think carefully, as long as you can bear the cost of the advantage of time and energy. Strolling to work now and then or using the stairwell rather than the lift a couple of times each week are prescribed for individuals to remain fit as a fiddle. Do you not need your brain to be fit too? Lay off the GPS now and again, and help your spatial and critical thinking abilities out. Keep it convenient, however, have a go at exploring barely first. Your brain will thank you for it.

5. Organization

What's more, that carries us to the last component to expand your psychological potential: Systems administration. What's extraordinary about this last goal is that on the off chance that you are doing the other four things; you are likely previously doing this also. If not, start. Right away

By systems administration with others—either through web-based media like Facebook or Twitter or in up close and personal cooperation—you are presenting yourself to the sorts of circumstances that will make destinations 1-4 a lot simpler to accomplish. By presenting yourself to new individuals, thoughts, and conditions, you are freeing yourself up to new freedoms for intellectual development. Being within the sight of others who might be outside of your nearby field gives you freedoms to see issues from another viewpoint or offer knowledge in manners that you had never considered. Learning is tied in with presenting yourself to new things and taking in that data in manners that are significant and special—organizing with others is an incredible method to get that going. I'm not in any event, going to get into the social advantages and passionate prosperity that is gotten from systems administration as a factor here, yet that is only an additional advantage.

Different creators have talked about the significance of gatherings and organizations for the headway of thoughts. If you are searching for approaches to search out novel circumstances, thoughts, conditions, and points of view, at that point organizing is the appropriate response. It would be really hard to execute this "Get More brilliant" regiment with making organizing an essential segment. The best thing about systems administration for everybody included advantages like Aggregate knowledge for success!

I recounted the tale about my customers with mental imbalance range problems? We should consider that briefly, considering all the other things we examined how to build your liquid insight. For what reason were those kids ready to accomplish at an undeniable level? It was not by some coincidence or marvel—it was because we fused these learning standards into their treatment program. While most other treatment suppliers were stuck in the "Errorless Learning" worldview and scarcely adjusted "Lovaas Procedures" of Applied Conduct Examination, we received and completely accepted a multimodal way to deal with instructing. We made the children battle to learn, we utilized the most inventive ways we could consider, and we tested them past what they appeared to be able to do—we set the bar exceptionally high. Yet, guess what? They outperformed that bar on numerous occasions and made me really accept that stunning things are conceivable if you have sufficient will and mental fortitude, and tirelessness to show yourself that way and stick with it. If those children with inabilities can carry on with this way of life of continually boosting their psychological potential, at that point so can you.

Also, I have a leaving question for you to consider too: If we have the entirety of this supporting information, showing that these training strategies and methods of moving toward learning can have a particularly significant beneficial outcome on intellectual development, for what reason aren't more treatment projects or educational systems receiving a portion of these procedures? I'd love to consider this to be the norm in educating, not the special case. How about we take a stab at something novel and shake up the teaching framework a tad, will we? We'd raise the aggregate level of intelligence to something else.

Intelligent is not just about the number of levels of math courses you've taken, how quickly you can settle a calculation or the number of vocabulary words you realize that are more than 6 characters. It's tied in with having the option to move toward another issue, perceive its significant segments, and settle it—at that point take that information acquired and put it towards addressing the following, more perplexing issue. It's about development and a creative mind and about having the option to put that to use to improve the world. This is the sort of knowledge that is significant and this is the kind of intelligent we ought to make progress toward.

CHAPTER TWO

FACTORS INFLUENCING INTELLIGENT QUOTIENT

DETERMINANT OF INTELLIGENT QUOTIENT

We as a whole realize that level of intelligence numbers say something regarding our insight, however, what precisely is the level of intelligence? A level of intelligence, shortened from IQ, is the absolute score got from state-sanctioned tests that action an individual's insight. The vast majority score between intelligence level 85 and level of intelligence 115, while geniuses score above the level of intelligence 130. Be that as it may, intelligence level is not totally dependable, and the numbers do not show all parts of an individual's knowledge. In any case, if you need to score more on your next level of intelligence test, perhaps doing a touch of brain practicing could help

How is knowledge estimated?

There are numerous approaches to gauge an individual's insight yet the most widely recognized of all is IQ (level of intelligence). In any case, there are banters with regards to the correct method of estimating insight, some differed that level of intelligence is the "right" approach to gauge one's knowledge.

How might you decide whether a kid has a below the norm level of intelligence?

A portion of the signs that decide whether a youngster has a below the norm intelligence level incorporate helpless social abilities according to a play-master circumstance, helpless dressing abilities, helpless taking care of abilities, helpless cleanliness, and self-care.

What are the signs that characterize a wise individual?

Insightful individuals love to teach themselves somehow. They are likewise versatile and liberal. Savvy individuals are additionally exceptionally incredulous and never reluctant to pose inquiries.

What are the approaches to thought of groundbreaking thoughts consistently?

There are various approaches to think of some extraordinary thoughts consistently remembering drawing in for perception meetings, mingling, understanding books, riding the web, keeping a diary, contemplating, utilizing organized activities, and much more.

How might reading support your insight?

Scientists discovered that reading a book gives you more information, accordingly, expands your insight as a rule. It additionally helps in improving insightful reasoning, jargon, and composing abilities.

How could instructive recordings improve your intelligence level?

Instructive video works with deduction, critical thinking abilities and helps with dominance acquiring, moves and energizes kids

What are the propensities that harm your brain?

Undesirable propensities that harm the mind incorporate burning through a lot of salt, lack of sleep, terrible hearing, a lot of food, dejection, and significantly more.

How might you animate your intellectual prowess?

On the off chance that you need to reestablish or animate your intellectual prowess, attempt basic exercises like working out, getting sufficient rest, and reading, retaining the superfluous, eating quality food sources, tuning in to or playing music and getting out of your usual range of familiarity.

How might you improve your concentration and core interest?

There are numerous approaches to improve your concentration and fixation. Be that as it may, the four significant approaches to do so incorporate getting enough cardio works out, drinking water, getting sufficient rest and squirming your toes to bring back your concentration immediately.

What is a brilliant game?

Keen games are those brain games, mental activities, or new exercises that make all the difference for your psyche.

What are the advantages of playing shrewd games?

According to research, grown-ups who for the most part play intellectually animating exercises are less inclined to create dementia by 63% contrasted with the individuals who seldom do so.

What are the various types of shrewd games?

The principal sorts of shrewd games incorporate crossword puzzles, Sudoku, mind riddles, brainteasers and mentally prepared platforms.

Would relaxation be able to improve your level of intelligence?

Indeed. Fundamentally, unwinding improves your insight as it permits you to zero in and fixate on things that need an essential reaction.

How might exercise and count calories influence your psychological well-being?

As indicated by research, what you eat really impacts your general capacity to recollect and the odds of creating dementia later on schedule.

FACTORS THAT CONTRIBUTE POSITIVELY TO YOUR INTELLIGENT QUOTIENT

The positive way of life decisions

The positive way of life decisions include:

- taking part consistently in active work
- .eating a decent eating regimen
- ..getting adequate rest
- Balancing school/work and different responsibilities
- making time for unwinding and recreation pursuits
- having great individual cleanliness
- recognizing the enthusiastic, social, and actual ramifications of sexual connections
- avoiding or limiting unsafe dangers, for example, smoking, drinking liquor, consuming medications

- Managing hazards in the more extensive climate, for example, street security and at home
- seeking information about or support for concerns, for example, companions, family, specialist, educator

FACTORS THAT CONTRIBUTE NEGATIVELY TO YOUR INTELLIGENT QUOTIENT

Long periods of driving and staring at the television lower intelligence level scores

Scientists have tracked down that driving for over two hours daily appears to consistently diminish insight.

The examination explored what inactive conduct means for mental aptitude. It discovered intelligence level scores fell quicker in moderately aged individuals who drove significant distances each day.

The individuals who drove more than a few hours daily ordinarily had lower intellectual prowess toward the beginning of the investigation, which continued declining all through and at a quicker rate than the individuals who did next to zero driving.

They find that routinely driving for more than a few hours daily is awful for your heart.

This exploration recommends it is awful for your brain as well, maybe because your psyche is less dynamic in those hours."

The scientists dissected the ways of life of more than 500,000 individuals matured somewhere in the range of 37 and 73 more than five years, during which they took insight and memory tests.

The 93,000 individuals who drove more than a few hours daily ordinarily had lower intellectual prowess toward the beginning of the examination which continued declining all through, at a quicker rate than the individuals who did practically zero driving.

A comparable outcome was additionally found for those sitting in front of the television for over three hours every day, who likewise had below intellectual prowess toward the beginning of the examination and which fell quicker over the course of the following five years. Nonetheless, this was not the situation for individuals who utilized a PC for a few hours out of every day, which recommends that PC use stimulatingly affects the mind.

The psychological decrease is quantifiable for more than five years since it can happen quickly in moderately aged and more seasoned individuals. This is related to way of life factors like smoking and a terrible eating routine — and now with time spent driving.

OTHER NEGATIVE LIFESTYLE CHOICES AND THE IMPLICATIONS

Making negative lifestyle choices can be active – something people do – or passive – something people choose not or neglect to do. They include:

- Detect any indications of brain fog(what might be compared to feeling sincerely troubled – it's practically how mind communicates pity past feelings) which could be brought about by activities like isolation, lockdowns, loss of expectation, and vulnerability

- Not doing enough physical activity

- being excessively stationary, for example, sitting or resting for extensive stretches

- having an unfortunate eating routine, for example eating excessively or excessively little, eating a lot of fat/sugar/salt

- Not getting sufficient rest or having whimsical rest designs

- Smoking

- abusing liquor, for example, drinking excessively as well as time after time

- misusing substances, for example ingesting medications, utilizing execution upgrading drugs, abusing remedy or over-the-counter medications

- self-hurting

- taking superfluous destructive dangers, for example having unprotected sex, rolling over as far as possible

- ignoring signs and side effects of sickness or enthusiastic strain

The impacts

A negative way of life influences the body and brain. The adverse consequences can be momentarily and long haul. They may likewise influence others, for instance, somebody's youngsters. For the most part, individuals are more roused to change their conduct to acquire positive advantages than to stay away from adverse consequences, particularly when the adverse consequences may not show up until far into what's to come.

CHAPTER THREE

WAYS AT WHICH YOU CAN IMPROVE YOUR INTELLIGENT QUOTIENT

Such countless ways and strategies by which you can improve your intelligence level of which you ought not to become weary of, The sum or level of your intelligence level says a great deal regarding you and will be to your advantage now and over the long haul.

1. Discover some new information

Memory strength is actually similar to strong strength. The more you use it, the more grounded it gets. However, you cannot lift a similar size weight each day and hope to get more grounded. You'll have to keep your brain continually tested. Acquiring ability is an amazing method to reinforce your brain's memory limit.

There are numerous exercises to browse, however above all, you'll need to discover something that constrains you out of your usual range of familiarity and orders your complete consideration.

Here are a few models:

- learn the use of musical instrument

- make pottery

- play mind games, similar to Sudoku or chess

- learn another kind of dance, similar to the tango

- learn another dialect

An examination from 2007 showed that communicating in more than one language can postpone the beginning of memory issues in individuals with dementia.

2. Rehash and recover

Any time you get familiar with another snippet of data, you're bound to intellectually record that data if it's rehashed. Redundancy builds up the associations we make between neurons. Rehash what you hear for all to hear. Have a go at utilizing it in a sentence. Record it and read it resoundingly.

In any case, the work does not stop there. Examination shows that straightforward redundancy is an inadequate learning instrument whenever utilized all alone. You'll have to sit down later and effectively attempt to recover the information without taking a look at where you recorded it. Testing yourself to recover the data is superior to continued consideration. Rehearsing recovery makes all the more long haul and significant learning encounters.

3. Attempt abbreviations, shortened forms, and memory aides

Memory helpers can be abbreviations, shortening melodies, or rhymes. Memory helpers have been tried since the 1960s as a successful technique for students. You've likely been shown a couple of mental helpers for recalling considerable records. For instance, the shades of the range can be recalled with the name ROY G. BIV (Red, Orange, Yellow, Green, Blue, Indigo, and Violet).

4. "Gathering" or "piece" data

Gathering or lumping alludes to the way toward partitioning recently educated data into pieces to deliver less, bigger lumps of data. For instance, you may have seen that it's a lot simpler to recollect a telephone number if the 10 digits are gathered into three separate lumps (for example 555-637-8299) instead of one long number (5556378299).

5. Develop a "mind royal residence"

The psyche royal residence method is regularly utilized by memory advocates. In this antiquated strategy, you make a visual and complex spot to store a bunch of recollections.

6. Utilize the entirety of your faculties

Another strategy of memory authority is that they do not simply depend on one sense to help hold data. All things considered, they relate data to different faculties, similar to tones, tastes, and scents.

7. Try not to dismiss to Google right

Current innovation has its place, yet shockingly has made us "intellectually sluggish." Before you go after your phone to ask Google, make a strong endeavor to recover the data with your brain. This cycle builds up the neural pathways in your mind.

8. Lose the GPS

Another regular misstep is depending on the GPS each time you drive. Scientists found in 2013 that depending on reaction procedures — like GPS — for route contracts a piece of our brain called the hippocampus, which is liable for spatial memory and moving data from the present moment to long haul memory. Helpless hippocampus wellbeing is related to dementia and memory decrease.

Except if you're completely lost, attempt to get to your objective thinking carefully rather than simply adhering to the directions on your GPS. Maybe use GPS to arrive, yet think carefully to get back home. Your brain will thank you for the additional test.

9. Keep yourself occupied

A bustling timetable can keep up your mind's rambling memory. One examination connected occupied timetables to better intellectual capacity. This examination, be that as it may, was restricted without anyone else announcing.

10. Stay coordinated

A coordinated individual makes some simpler memories recalling. Agendas are one acceptable device for associations. Physically recording your agenda (rather than doing it electronically) likewise improves the probability that you'll recall what you've recorded.

11. Rest on a customary timetable

Hit the hay simultaneously consistently and get up simultaneously every morning. Make an effort not to break your daily practice at the end of the week. This can significantly improve rest quality.

12. Keep away from visual screens before bed

The blue light discharged by phones, television, and PC screens represses the creation of melatonin, a chemical that controls your rest wake cycle (circadian mood). An inadequately managed rest cycle can truly negatively affect rest quality.

Without enough rest and rest, the neurons in our brains become exhausted. They cannot, at this point facilitate data, making it harder to get to recollections. Approximately an hour before sleep time, turn off your gadgets and permit your mind to loosen up.

13. Eat a greater amount of these food sources:

Diets like the Mediterranean eating regimen, Run (dietary ways to deal with hypertension), and the Psyche diet (Mediterranean-Run mediation for the neurodegenerative postponement) share a couple of things for all intents and purpose. This incorporates their capacity to improve memory and decrease the danger of Parkinson's and Alzheimer's sickness.

These eating regimens center on eating:

- Plant-based food sources, particularly green, verdant vegetables and berries

- Whole grains

- Legumes

- Nuts
- Chicken or turkey
- Olive oil or coconut oil
- Herbs and flavors
- Fatty fish, like salmon and sardines
- Red wine, with some restraint

Greasy fish are a rich sources of omega-3 unsaturated fats. Omega-3s assume a significant part in building mind and nerve cells. They're fundamental for learning and memory and have been appeared to defer intellectual decay.

14. Eat less of these food sources:

Defenders of the Mediterranean and Psyche counts calories say to keep away from the accompanying food sources:

- Sugar
- processed food varieties
- Butter

- Red meat
- fried food varieties
- Salt
- Cheese

Sugar and fat have been connected to impeded memory. A new report in people tracked down that an eating regimen high in fats and sugars — regular in a Western eating routine — debilitates hippocampal memory. Notwithstanding, the examination depended on polls and overviews, which may not be as precise.

15. Keep away from specific prescriptions

While you should in any case take your prescriptions recommended by your physician, make sure to adhere to your primary care physician's guidelines for dietary and way of life changes as well.

A few remedies, similar to statins for elevated cholesterol, have been related to cognitive decline and "brain haze." Getting more fit and eating better may likewise assume a part in treating elevated cholesterol.

Different drugs/prescriptions that may influence memory negatively include:

- Antidepressants
- Anti-uneasiness drugs
- Hypertension drugs
- sleeping pills
- metformin

Discuss with your PCP(primary care physician) about how to deal with your ailments so that you do not need to depend on a remedy for eternity. In case you're stressed over what a prescription may mean for your memory, converse with your PCP about your alternatives.

16. Get physical

Running, cycling, yoga, and strength preparing would all be able to make you more astute in all honesty. Exploration including neuro-imaging directed in the previous decade shows that actual exercise improves psychological wellbeing and even upgrades the working of mind areas liable for controlling your intellectual cycles. Exercise is accepted to tweak metabolic components that help the brain working. Exercise is likewise said to improve our DNA utilizing epigenetic systems. However, to lay it out plainly, the expanded oxygen consumption, better sustenance, chemical delivery, synapse changes, and different things occurring during exercise impact our mind on the atomic level and this clearly makes you more intelligent.

Practicing has been appeared to have psychological advantages. It improves oxygen and supplement conveyance to the body and assists with making new cells in the mind which are fundamental for memory stockpiling. Exercise particularly expands the number of cells in the hippocampus.

There's no requirement for the activity to be difficult. Strolling, for instance, is an extraordinary decision.

17. Oversee pressure

At the point when you're focused, your body discharges pressure chemicals like cortisol. Cortisol has appeared to extraordinarily debilitate the brains memory interaction, particularly our capacity to recover long-haul recollections. Stress and misery have even been appeared in creature studies to contract the brain.

18. Mingle

People are social animals. Examination shows that a solid emotionally supportive network is fundamental to our passion and brain wellbeing. One investigation from 2007 found that individuals with dynamic public activities had the slowest memory decrease. Only 10 minutes of conversing with someone else were appeared to improve memory.

21. Reduction in liquor consumption

Moderate utilization of liquor may surely positively affect memory; however, remember that moderate methods only one beverage for ladies and two for men every day.

Drinking beyond that can hurt your capacity to hold data.

22. Meditation

There's mounting proof for the medical advantages of reflection. Studies show that reflection improves a few intellectual capacities, similar to center, fixation, memory, and learning. Reflection may really revamp the brain and support more associations between synapses.

23. Appreciate nature

Getting out into nature is extraordinarily significant for our passion and actual wellbeing. Appreciating nature can even be viewed as a type of contemplation. One 2008 investigation tracked down that a stroll in a recreation center improved memory and consideration contrasted with strolling in a city.

Similarly, every day planting brings down your danger of dementia by 36%, as indicated by one 2006 examination.

24. Shed the additional weight

Individuals with more greasy tissue will in general have less water than individuals with less greasy tissue. Overweight and obese individuals likewise have less brain tissue. The more overweight you are, the more your brain is probably going to have a difficult time concentrating and processing information.

Our memory is an expertise, and very much like different abilities, it tends to be improved with pursuing and solid generally speaking routines. You can begin little. For instance, pick another provoking action to learn, join a couple of moments of activity into your day, keep a rest plan, and eat a couple of more green vegetables, fish, and nuts.

The following time you need to read for a test, attempt one of the procedures recommended by memory support, such as lump, mind royal residences, or recovery.

Discuss with your PCP on the off chance that you notice that you're committing a lot more errors than expected or experience difficulty finishing straightforward everyday assignments, such as cooking or cleaning.

25. Riddles and games

You'll discover crossword riddles and games like Sudoku frequently being prescribed for those considering how to improve their memory, yet do they work? All things considered, an examination that was distributed in PLoS One intended to discover only that by allowing youthful grown-ups to mess around Tetris and Cerebrum, it influence different parts of their psychological capacities, including their intelligence level. What the examination found was that these kinds of games increase chief capacities, working memory, and preparing speed however not an individual's intelligence level. This means alleged mind games only exercise a few spaces of mental working yet not others. All in all, on the off chance that you play a game that improves your memory may not really improve your painting or playing the piano.

26. Try not to depend on your gadgets to such an extent

Our PCs and different gadgets have gotten progressively effective in doing the vast majority of our work for us. While this is, in one way, something to be thankful for, it might likewise make our brain somewhat lazy and dependent. Rehearsing your mathematical abilities by doing your computations now and again and killing spell-check when composing, You'll most likely discover numerous changes in your everyday life to rehearse straightforward math and spelling expertise, for example, with your financial exercises while taking care of your bills when assessment documenting, messaging or shopping for food. Try to utilize what you've realized in school in your regular daily existence, so every one of those hours you've spent contemplating does not go to squander.

27. Starve your mind

This may appear to be irrational; however, abandoning nourishment for quite a while may help your brain stay sharp over the long haul. For example, continuous fasting, which includes abandoning nourishment for around 16 hours and eating your standard dinner toward the finish of a fasting period was found to make the brain stronger to harm. This training will likewise expand the number of new neurons to more discoveries. Thus, avoid eating food for while to help your intellectual prowess, and do not eat any food varieties all things being equal – yet for a brief timeframe, obviously.

28. Keep a diary

Composing diaries is an incredible method to think about your life and express your emotions through the composed word. However, the training can likewise help you upgrade basic intuition as indicated by certain specialists. All in all, specialists concur that diary composing improves intelligent reasoning which is something you would not see being tried in intelligence level tests. All things considered, keeping a diary will grow your vocabulary, give an enthusiastic outlet, and even assist with depression. Then again, you can begin publishing content to a blog which is basically a type of journal-style composing. The social part of writing for a blog will likewise push you to your intellectual abilities since you'll need to make your entrances respectable.

29. Get familiar with ability

Learning ought not to be something you only do in school. Get familiar with a specialty, another dialect, or take up another side interest. Figuring out how to do new things will keep your psyche dynamic and animate spaces of your psychological working that may have been ignored and remember that variety is key. All intelligence level tests basically check your capacity to discover answers for new circumstances. Since mastering ability will necessitate that you explore through new data, you'll become better at critical thinking thus. What's more, if you have a feeling that you would not figure out how to do new things, do not let that hold you back from utilizing your full intellectual abilities. An examination distributed quite recently in Investigations in Wellbeing Innovation, and Informatics found that your certainty levels and demeanor assume a gigantic part in the ability to master new abilities.

30. Figure out how to play an instrument

There's a developing assemblage of examination connecting instrument playing to more noteworthy psychological capacities in the two youngsters and grown-ups. Some research distributed in the Boondocks in Brain research clarifies that perusing and playing music is an intricate movement including engine and tactile performing multiple tasks. Other than that, playing music strongly affects your feelings, and this also can decidedly influence your intellectual abilities. The article being referred to covers an examination that contrasted the impacts of piano learning and a benchmark group and tracked down that the piano gathering performed better in Stroop tests.

31. Improve your social abilities

Therapists have likewise found that there is a solid connection between's social abilities and level of intelligence scores. Significantly, we likewise realize that social abilities can be educated. So improving your social abilities will thus build your level of intelligence score. Social abilities are essentially the comprehension of a small bunch of numerical connections between ideas or items, for example, things are equivalent to different things, pretty much than different things, inverse to different things, etc. They likewise incorporate connections like prior and then afterward or that one thing is contained by another. Additionally, having a solid handle on the connections between and in addition to other things has been appeared to improve thinking and critical thinking abilities. Truth be told, these social abilities are presently being known as the structure squares of knowledge by clinicians in the field of Social Casing Hypothesis.

32. Advance your language

It is normally acknowledged that coming from a language-rich climate will build an individual's scholarly intuition. In any case, I'll bet you did not realize that for those that do not come from such a climate, you can peruse broadly to build your vocabulary and compensate for that "shortfall" in your common habitat. Exploration demonstrates that having a solid comprehension of language will assist you with numerous psychological errands and for sure with regular daily existence. Expanding your vocabulary by perusing will build your comprehension of language in a more broad sense. Additionally, keep a decent word reference. At the point when you run over words that you do not have a clue or are inexperienced with, do not be reluctant to "find it".

33. Appeal to the specialists

Now and again you cannot discover the responses to the inquiries in your psyche on the Web or from reference books, when that occurs; it's an ideal opportunity to ask the specialists. Simply ensure that the specialists you are asking for are really educated and proficient sources. There is a lot of data out there that is essentially wrong, so consistently search for logical proof sponsorship up any "realities".

34. Have a development mentality

It is a moderately late disclosure that your mentality matters on a passionate level, yet additionally a physiological level. Accepting that you can learn more will improve your exhibition in any learning climate. Persevering with undertakings in any event, when they are troublesome will assist you with getting to the end goal.

35. Step outside your usual range of familiarity

Examination shows that we can expand our brain's working by driving ourselves to learn things that are outside of our present range of abilities. So figure out how to play music, to move or evaluate another dialect. Interestingly, you are programming your brain in another way and this manner growing your mind's neural organizations. Keeping your mind fit and dynamic is particularly significant as you enter a more seasoned adulthood.

OTHER BASIC APPROACHES TO IMPROVE YOUR LEVEL OF INTELLIGENCE

The accompanying data realistic outwardly traces approaches to improve your level of intelligence, including:

- Come up with 10 thoughts consistently

- Follow your inquiries

- Play argumentative third party

- Watch instructive recordings rather than TV

- Read the newspaper, articles, journals and other related works

- Check in with your number one information sources

- Share what you learn with others

- Apply what you learn

- Start a "Quit Doing" list

- Write down what you realize

- Stimulate your psyche
- Take online courses
- Talk to somebody you discover intriguing
- Subscribe to feeds of intriguing data
- Play "brilliant" games
- Use an expression of-the-day application
- Do something alarming
- Explore new regions
- Hang out with individuals who are more intelligent than you
- Set to the side some an ideal opportunity to sit idle
- Adopt a beneficial diversion you can rehearse every day
- Memory exercises.
- Management control exercises.
- Visuospatial thinking exercises.

- Relational abilities.
- Musical instruments.
- New dialects.
- Frequent perusing.
- Continued instruction.

CHAPTER FOUR

THE SIGNIFICANCE OF MENTAL WELLNESS

Keeping your brain fit as a fiddle

Actual wellness gets a lot of consideration and in light of current circumstances. A solid body can forestall conditions like coronary illness and diabetes, and assist you with keeping up freedom as you age.

Mental wellness is similarly pretty much as significant as actual wellness, and should not be disregarded. Counting mental adroitness practices into your everyday schedule can assist you with receiving the rewards of a more honed mind and a better body for quite a long time to come.

Mental wellness implies keeping your brain and enthusiastic wellbeing fit as a fiddle does not mean preparing for "brain Olympics" or an intelligence level test. It alludes to a progression of activities that help you:

- slow down
- decompress
- boost a hailing memory

Mind body association

It's nothing unexpected that the more you help your body, the more you help your mind. Active work builds the progression of oxygen to your mind. It additionally expands the number of endorphins, the "vibe great" synthetic compounds, in your brain. Consequently, it's not astounding that individuals who are fit as a fiddle likewise will in general appreciate a more elevated level of mental readiness.

Taking part in an incredible actual exercise can help you fight gloom and gain a more inspirational point of view. It's additionally an extraordinary method to beat pressure, which can hurt you intellectually and truly.

Mental exercise is comparably helpful. According to an examination by neuroscientists, certain memory preparing activities can build "liquid intelligent," the capacity to reason and tackle new issues.

While practice is useful for the mind and the body, so is contemplation. Reflection, related to different techniques, is an effective method to treat sadness. Quieting the mind permits you to settle in a more loosened-up manner.

Advantages of mental wellness

At the point when you hit the bed in the wake of a difficult day, your body starts to unwind. However, the mind does not generally follow.

Perception can help you frequently accomplish a feeling of serenity through symbolism, the way toward imagining a peaceful scene or area. This training can decrease strain in both your body and your psyche by testing neurons in the less prevailing space of your mind.

The less predominant side of your brain is simply the territory that controls sentiments certainty and idealism. At the point when you consider some different options from your day-by-day stresses, you increase action in the neural designs of that space of your brain.

At last, perception can support your passionate prosperity and makes you settle down intellectually.

Become intellectually fit

Keeping your brain intellectually fit is not just about as troublesome as preparing for a long-distance race, yet it's a decent relationship. You can add mental activities to the numerous exercises you as of now perform, for example,

- daydreaming
- finding humor throughout everyday life

You may attempt the accompanying ways to deal with increasing your psychological wellness.

Quit multitasking

You may imagine that performing multiple tasks empowers you to complete more things without a moment's delay; however, it really makes a larger number of issues than it tackles. Zeroing in on each errand in turn will improve your fixation and assist you with being more gainful.

Be positive with yourself

The positive assertion is one road to expanded mental capability.

Attestation or decidedly discussing with you yourself includes reinforcing neural pathways to bring your self-assurance, prosperity and fulfillment to a more elevated level.

To begin, make a rundown of your great characteristics. Advise yourself that you do not need to be awesome. Set objectives for what you need to improve and begin little to try not to get overpowered.

Take a stab at something other than what's expected New encounters can likewise show you the way to mental wellness. You can fit new methodologies into your everyday life in an assortment of ways:

- Try new food sources.

- Try better approaches to achieve routine assignments.

- Travel to new places.

- Take another approach to work or the supermarket.

According to studies directed by a board of neurosurgeons which shows that keeping your brain dynamic builds its essentialness. Doing new things in new manners seems to help hold synapses and associations. It might even create new synapses. Basically, breaking out of your routine can help keep your mind stay solid.

Take the time

Mental wellness does not need to take up a great deal of your time. Putting in no time limit on it consistently can help you feel much improved and think all the more unmistakably. Recollect that unwinding and perception are similarly as significant in a psychological exercise as the more vigorous exercises, for example, memory activities or game-playing. Have a go at adding each or two exercises in turn to your psychological exercise, for example,

- relaxing
- visualizing
- affirming
- Memory work-out
- Build Solid connections:

The absolute initial phase in building a solid relationship and sound connection with your loved ones is to talk. The more you talk with them, the more you moved from stress which gets you far from Mental Pressure. A solid family remaining by you is all that you require battling all chances of mental challenges throughout everyday life.

CHAPTER FIVE

THE CONNECTION AMONG DEPRESSION AND COGNITIVE DECLINE

Managing depression can be an exceptionally overpowering encounter. There is a great deal of passionate agony that you might be encountering. You might be overpowered with anguish, trouble, disgrace, or blame and you may even feel sad. Also, there are numerous actual indications of gloom that you could be encountering like migraines, constant agony, exhaustion, and processing issues. But on the other hand, there's another result of sadness that numerous individuals are new to. There's been discovered to join among sorrow and cognitive decline.

WHAT EXPERTS ARE SAYING

Specialists in one 2013 investigation found that individuals with depression could not distinguish objects on a screen that were indistinguishable or like an item they had seen already. As indicated by analysts, this proposes that memory can be reduced because of melancholy. Specialists in a recent report arrived at a comparable resolution. They inferred that downturn may cause momentary cognitive decline

At the point when Cognitive decline Prompts Gloom

IS THERE AN ASSOCIATION AMONG DESPONDENCY AND COGNITIVE DECLINE?

It's simple for individuals to comprehend that those that are encountering cognitive decline due to age or illnesses like Alzheimer's could encounter depression too. We can fold our heads over the possibility that realizing that you are battling with your memory can make you go into different indications of sadness. It's a major change in life when managing actual issues and it's normal for those that have an ongoing medical issue to encounter sadness.

That does not imply that these sicknesses are straightforwardly identified with depression, yet just that when individuals are encountering various afflictions, they might be bound to encounter manifestation of despondency also. In any case, this is not the lone connection between cognitive decline and discouragement.

HOW DOES DEPRESSION CAUSE COGNITIVE DECLINE?

There was a broad examination which led to explore the effect of despondency on memory. They tried just about 100 grown-ups to discover what their outcomes would do to an example detachment test. The investigation tracked down that the higher the level of the downturn score of the member, the lower score they got on the example division test.

The scientists accept that when somebody is encountering discouragement, they likewise experience more significant levels of memory obstruction than they would if they were not encountering manifestations of misery.

Memory obstruction is the point at which an individual cannot take in and review new data in light of past circumstances or encounters that they are managing. In the case of despondency, since somebody is encountering changes in their idea design, energy levels, and inspiration, they cannot actually take in and review new data the very way that they would do for something else. It might be said, they're not ready to focus like they would on the off chance that they were not discouraged.

After the consequences of the investigation, the scientists accept that a cycle called design division is harmed when somebody is encountering depression. This cycle or interaction is the thing that permits individuals to deal or cope with various circumstances and things that are like one another. With this cycle not working effectively, somebody with gloom cannot remember the subtleties of the circumstance that would assist them with isolating it from whatever else. It might be said, recollections mix because the downturn does not permit them to get sufficient various things to isolate them from one another. So there's nothing that stands apart from them about the data that makes it simple for them to review.

What's more, scientists tracked down that the hippocampus, which is liable for memory has a diminished development rate in circumstances of depression. The hippocampus is additionally in the space of the mind that develops new synapses. Consequently, when somebody is living with gloom, the genuine capacity of their brain to take in and review new data is contrarily affected.

DIFFERENT REASONS FOR COGNITIVE DECLINE

Different reasons you may encounter cognitive decline can incorporate the following:

- Normal age-related cognitive decline is normal and reasonable. One illustration of this is failing to remember where you put your glasses yet recalling later in the day.

- Alzheimer's infection is the most well-known type of dementia. It can cause reformist, hopeless mind harm, and cognitive decline.

- Mild psychological debilitation can modify thinking abilities and ultimately progress to Alzheimer's infection or different types of dementia.

- Minor head injury or injury can trigger slight memory issues, regardless of whether you did or did not pass out.

- Forgetfulness is an expected result of specific prescriptions.

- Brain tumors or mind diseases can influence your memory or trigger dementia-like indications.

- Vitamin B-12 insufficiency can make issues with your memory. This is because you're not keeping up solid nerve cells and red platelets.

- Alcoholism or medication misuse can weaken your psychological state and capacities. This can likewise happen when liquor cooperates with prescriptions.

- Hypothyroidism eases back your digestion, which can prompt memory issues and different issues with deduction.

- Brain or nerve harm brought about by sicknesses like Parkinson's infection or various scleroses can mess memory up. A recent report found that individuals with depression have more danger of building up Parkinson's infection.

Electroconvulsive treatment (ECT) can cause cognitive decline. ECT adjusts mind science, which can switch the side effects of sorrow and other dysfunctional behaviors. On the off chance that you have ECT, your primary care physician will perform it while you're under broad sedation. During ECT, your PCP sends little electric flows through your mind, setting off a concise seizure. Individuals can encounter disarray and transient cognitive decline after getting ECT medicines.

IS COGNITIVE DECLINE AND SADNESS TREATABLE?

Fortunately, both cognitive decline and sadness are treatable. In case you're encountering cognitive decline that is brought about by discouragement you can make a move to improve it. On the off chance that your cognitive decline is really the after effect of another illness or turmoil which probably would not be conceivable. However, assuming discouragement is the place where it's beginning, there are things that you can do to improve it.

There is a drug that has been known to decidedly affect those that are encountering cognitive decline and gloom. This drug is regularly utilized in patients that have Alzheimer's, you can discuss this with your physician. Notwithstanding, assuming cognitive decline is a side effect or consequence of your downturn, there are different things that you can do to improve your memory too. Your cognitive decline should not be an enduring result that you experience due to sadness.

A few specialists have been striving to grow new types of drug intensifies that would attempt to help turn around the harm of cognitive decline brought about by despondency.

Treating the Reason

If your cognitive decline is brought about by depression, you should remember that you need to treat the reason for the issue. Simply treating the cognitive decline would not be only about as successful as figuring out how to defeat the downturn that is causing it.

In case you're encountering cognitive decline and sorrow, you should converse with psychological well-being expert . A specialist will actually want to help you work through large numbers of your side effects of gloom, learn if there is where it is originating from, and learn methodologies that you can use to conquer it.

Discouragement is a treatable emotional wellness condition. It is not something that you need to simply keep living with whenever you have been analyzed. Various types of treatment are accessible, so the sooner that you follow up on finding support, the sooner you will actually want to stop the cognitive decline that you are encountering.

If you accept that you are encountering indications of cognitive decline and do not know whether you have sadness or not, at that point it's essential to converse with clinical experts, examine what you are eating, your environment or check your lifestyle. To decide how to address the cognitive decline, it will be essential to figure out the thing causing it. While depression is one of the reasons for cognitive decline there are numerous different things that very well may be identified with it. Getting the appropriate finding is the initial step to having the option to find support.

ADAPTING TO COGNITIVE DECLINE

Encountering cognitive decline could be a terrifying inclination. Particularly if you do not know whether it will be long haul or not, notwithstanding, while at the same time working at treating whatever is causing the cognitive decline there are some adapting tips that you can use to improve your everyday life.

Something you can do is getting yourself coordinated. The less mess that you need to manage at work or home the simpler it will be to monitor the things that you really need. It's likewise useful to ensure you're utilizing a schedule to follow any of the occasions or arrangements that you need to join in. It's too simple when you're managing depression to hear something and not spotlighting on it enough that you fail to remember what it is you've dedicated to. Ensure that you are putting everything down on a schedule. If you can, utilize a schedule on your telephone or another gadget so it can caution you with an alert when you have someplace that you should be.

It's additionally useful to utilize notes to help yourself to remember whatever you need to recall. This could be keeping notes by your telephone of individuals that you need to call, putting a note on your schedule on the off chance that you need to take care of a bill, or making a plan for the day for your day to help you understand what undertakings you should be centered around on achieving. At the point when you're battling with sorrow, it tends to be hard to need to do anything so you need to create it as simple as possible to know where your consideration should be going.

It can likewise be useful to keep a diary during this time or simply ensure that you're recording things. The demonstration of recording things on paper rather than basically keeping them electronically has been found to assist you with submitting that data to your memory. Toward the end of your day requires a couple of moments to review the occasion of your day in any discussions that you've had. This can assist you with bettering recollect what you need to.

Similarly, as with gloom, it's essential to keep up great self-care when working with cognitive decline. Getting sufficient rest, staying with a solid eating regimen and getting sufficient exercise every week can go far in improving your psychological well-being and actual wellbeing. I never wonder whether or not to connect with an advisor for extra assistance and to learn additional adapting techniques that you can use to defeat your downturn and cognitive decline.

WHAT CAN BE DONE TO PROTECT COGNITION?

Fortunately, the effect on cognizance from depression can be brief (and is commonly accepted to influence simply transient memory abilities), albeit rehashed scenes of depression can prompt all the more dependable intellectual medical problems. As well as looking for treatment and other proper medicines from a confided in psychological wellness professional, there are a few things individuals who are encountering sorrow can really do to secure their intellectual wellbeing, Adding more food sources with omega-3 unsaturated fats can help support your serotonin levels, and make sure to eat even dinners and to drink a lot of water. This may sound fundamental, yet these mind-solid propensities can help normally produce a greater amount of those immeasurably significant synapses that the brain needs to work appropriately.

What you cannot deny is that weakness is an admonition sign to make changes. It is imperative to allow yourself to rest when required and begin to take a look at your sleep time propensities and how you fuel your body with supplements and the required food sources during the day.

Although, it is hard to do when in a burdensome state, exercising is another incredible mindset improving action for the brain. On the off chance that you can gather up the energy for 30 minutes of oxygen-consuming activity, it can have a significant effect.

A few groups have by and by discovered journaling and reflection to be extraordinarily gainful to both their downturn indications and their memory. There are around 5000 reasons why I implore the use of diary consistently yet it can likewise truly help our memory banks, I additionally do week after week, month to month, quarterly, and yearly surveys of my phone photographs, my excursions, the highs and lows of those time spans, and so on [and] that has unquestionably helped also. Concerning reflection, it gives lucidity. At the point when I'm sensible, I recollect my days and discussions such a great deal better.

None of these ways of life changes on their own will mysteriously an individual's downturn, yet taken couple with different endeavors—like talk or light treatment—these things can truly assist individuals with dealing with their downturn side effects. For certain individuals, the drug is important to reestablish sound brain science, and there is no disgrace about that! We should take a look at all of these arrangements—diet, work out, treatment, medicine—basically as instruments in the tool stash."

As far as it concerns her, her all-encompassing methodology has truly assisted her better with dealing with her downturn manifestations— including her memory issues. I've in every case only imagine I had a terrible memory. However, I'm three years past the most exceedingly terrible of it, and my memory is such a great deal better! My entire life is better, yet certainly my memory as well.

CHAPTER SIX

THE PLACE OF NUTRITION

Adopting a solid eating routine is acceptable yet now and again which food sources are by and large sound? How would you know them and in what sum are they beneficial for you?

Nourishment assumes a fundamental part in brain work and remaining sharp into your brilliant years. Certain food varieties improve memory; do some incredible things in lessening aggravation in the brain. We will analyze these food varieties in this chapter

Here are the best brain food sources that improve memory and mental ability:

1. Water

The principal sustenance or substance that your mind needs are water, ensure the water you're taken contains a low or zero measure of acidic elements yet Alkaline based with a few minerals most particularly zinc and magnesium. You've presumably heard that up to 60% of the all-out human grown-up body is water. Notwithstanding, you probably have not heard that the brain and heart are made out of 73% water, and the lungs sit at about 83% water, If your mind is around 3/4 water, and you are dried out, do you figure how it will perform?

Odds are that a dried-out human will not arriving at top performance on the following physical science or math test, or anything besides!

While most suggestions center around drinking 8 glasses of water a day, new examinations have uncovered that may not generally be the best principle to follow. To know when you ought to drink water and which amount, tune in to your body. Your mind and body have developed modern procedures to advise you when you need water.

At the point when the mind identifies an absence of water, it will convey messages that reveal to you you're de-hydrated. When you start to feel like that, begin drinking water until you feel satisfied. Your body realizes how to really focus on its brain wellbeing, so trust it!

2. Nuts and Seeds

One investigation had the option to interface higher admissions of Vitamin E with the anticipation of intellectual decay.

If you need to up your admission of Vitamin E, Nuts like walnuts and almonds are acceptable sources. Cashews and sunflower seeds additionally contain an amino acid that decreases pressure by boosting serotonin levels.

Walnut even look like the mind, simply if you fail to remember the relationship, they are an extraordinary source of omega-3 unsaturated fats, which additionally improve your psychological extent.

3. Blueberries

With regards to food sources that improve memory, blueberries have been appeared to bring to the table incredible mind benefits and are extraordinary memory-upgrading food varieties. One examination on more established grown-ups tracked down that the individuals who drank blueberry juice showed improvement in matched partner learning and word list review.

When contrasted with different products of the soil, blueberries have the most noteworthy measure of cell reinforcements (particularly flavonoids), yet strawberries, raspberries, and blackberries are likewise brimming with brain benefits that can offer improved perception.

4. Tomatoes

Tomatoes are stuffed brimming with the cell reinforcement lycopene, which has appeared to help secure against free-radicals harm, most eminently found in dementia patients. Tomatoes are additionally extraordinary because you can sneak them into pretty much anything, including sauces, plates of mixed greens, and meat dishes by the way.

5. Broccoli

While all green veggies are significant and rich in cell reinforcements and vitamin C, broccoli is a super food even among these solid decisions.

Since your brain utilizes such a lot of fuel (it's just 3% of your body weight yet utilizes something like 17% of your energy), it is more defenseless against free-radicals harm, and cell reinforcements help kill this danger, such countless food varieties that improve memory incorporate these cancer prevention agents.

Broccoli is stuffed brimming with cell reinforcements, is notable as an incredible disease warrior, and is additionally brimming with vitamin K, which is known to upgrade psychological capacity. In particular, vitamin K is "associated with sphingolipids digestion, a class of lipids that partake in the multiplication, separation, and endurance of synapses."

6. Food varieties Rich in Fundamental Unsaturated fats

Your mind is the fattiest organ (not including the skin) in the human body and is made out of 60% fat. That implies that your brain needs fundamental unsaturated fats like DHA and EPA to fix and develop neurotransmitters related to memory.

The body does not normally deliver fundamental unsaturated fats, so we should get them into our eating regimen.

Eggs, flax, and sleek fish like salmon, sardines, mackerel, and herring are extraordinary characteristic sources of these incredible unsaturated fats. Eggs additionally contain choline, which is a vital structure block for the synapse acetylcholine, to help you review data and concentrate.

7. Soy

Soy, alongside numerous other entire food varieties referenced here, is brimming with proteins that trigger synapses related to memory. Soy protein confine is a concentrated type of protein that can be found in powder, fluid, or supplement structure.

Soy is significant for improving memory and mental adaptability, so pour soy milk over your oat and appreciate the advantages.

8. Dark Chocolate

With regards to chocolate the darker the better, attempt to focus on in any event 70% cocoa. This yummy pastry is rich in flavonol cancer prevention agents, which increases the bloodstream to the brain and safeguard synapses from maturing, making it perhaps the most delicious food that improves memory.

9. Food varieties Rich in Vitamin: Vitamin B, Folic Acid, Iron

Some incredible food varieties to acquire brain boosting B vitamins, folic acid and iron are kale, chard, spinach, and other dull, verdant greens. B6, B12, and folic acid can diminish levels of homocysteine in the blood. Homocysteine increments are found in patients with a psychological disability like Alzheimer's and those with a high danger of stroke.

Studies showed that when a gathering of older patients with gentle intellectual debilitation was given high dosages of B6, B12, and folic acid, there was a huge decrease in brain shrinkage contrasted with a comparable fake treatment bunch.

Different sources of vitamin B are liver, eggs, soybeans, lentils, and green beans. Iron additionally speeds up mind work via conveying oxygen. On the off chance that your brain does not get sufficient oxygen, it can back off and individuals can encounter trouble concentrating, decreased acumen, and a more limited capacity to focus.

To get more iron in your eating regimen, eat lean meats, beans, and iron-invigorated grains. Vitamin C aids in iron ingestion, so remember the organic products!

10. Food sources Rich in Zinc

Zinc has continually shown its significance as an incredible supplement in memory building and thinking, so food sources that improve memory will frequently incorporate this significant component. This mineral directs interchanges among neurons and the hippocampus.

Zinc is saved inside nerve cells, with the most elevated focuses found in the hippocampus, the piece of the brain answerable for higher learning capacity and memory.

Some incredible sources of zinc are pumpkin seeds, liver, nuts, and peas.

11. Ginkgo Biloba

This spice has been used for quite a long time in Eastern culture and is most popular for its memory-boosting muscle. It can build the bloodstream in the mind by widening vessels, expanding oxygen supply, and eliminating free extremists.

Be that as it may, do not expect results for the time being: this may require half a month to develop in your framework before you see enhancements.

12. Green and Dark Tea

Exploration proposes that both green and dark tea forestall the breakdown of acetylcholine—a key compound engaged with memory and ailing in Alzheimer's patients. This makes them incredible food varieties that improve memory.

The two groups seem to have a similar impact on Alzheimer's sickness as numerous medications are used to battle the disease; however, green tea wins out as its belongings last an entire week, versus dark tea, which just keeps going the day.

13. Sage and Rosemary

Both of these incredible spices have been appeared to build memory and mental clearness, and reduce mental exhaustion in different examinations. Pair a portion of the above food varieties that invigorate the mind with these stunning spices in soups, servings of mixed greens, or even in teas!

14. Krill Oil/Fish Oils

I've indicated krill oil here; in any case, you are free to take any type of excellent fish oil supplement as a brain enhancer, another model being Alaskan wild salmon oil. I would, obviously, recommend cooked fish rather than supplementation. In any case, you can profit from both.

Omega-3 unsaturated fats are polyunsaturated fats liable for the majority of the mind and emotional wellness,

Fish oil fundamentally contains two sorts of omega-3 unsaturated fats — EPA and DHA. These unsaturated fats are basic for ordinary mind capacity and improvement all through all phases of life. EPA and DHA assume significant parts in building up an infant's brain.

Indeed, a few investigations have connected pregnant ladies' fish admission or fish oil use with expanded scores for their youngsters on the trial of knowledge and brain work in youth. These EPA/DHA unsaturated fats are additionally essential for the upkeep of typical mind work all through life. They are bountiful in the cell films of synapses, protecting cell layer wellbeing and working with correspondence between synapses.

Cooked or barbecued fish or fish oils may likewise improve mind work in individuals with memory issues, like people with Alzheimer's sickness or other psychological debilitations.

Fish Oil Supplement would be a pleasant alternative.

In case you're feeling absent-minded, it very well maybe because of an absence of rest or some different reasons, including hereditary qualities, level of actual work, and way of life, and ecological variables. Nonetheless, there's no uncertainty that diet additionally assumes a part in mental wellbeing.

The best menu for supporting memory and mind work urges a great bloodstream to the brain—

similar to what you'd eat to feed and secure your heart. Exploration tracking down the Mediterranean Eating regimen may help to continue keeping maturing minds sharp and a developing collection of proof connections food sources like those in the Mediterranean eating routine with better intellectual capacity, memory, and sharpness.

15. Matured food varieties

The most recent exploration shows that the microbes in our guts and stomach-related plot can straightforwardly affect our minds, as indicated by a nutritionist "A few researchers would go similarly as considering our gut our second brain in light of these examinations.

The best food varieties for your brain are those that are high in acceptable Probiotic Microorganisms. Matured food varieties like kimchi, sauerkraut, kefir, and miso are extraordinary alternatives for dealing with your mind through your gut. They're likewise too delicious."

16. Brilliant Foods grown from the ground

Cell reinforcements extinguish free radicals inside our body and decrease irritation. Aggravation in the brain can build the danger of dementia, Alzheimer's, and Parkinson's illness and it additionally expands the danger for sadness, as indicated by clinical specialists. "Fill your plate with bright products of the soil at every dinner. 'Eat the rainbow' is not only a snappy expression. The shade of various foods grown from the ground connotes their cell reinforcement content so when we eat a wide range of tones, we are getting in a wide range of cancer prevention agents in our body, all of which have diverse medical advantages."

.17. Turmeric

An antiquated spice generally utilized in Indian cooking and culinary, turmeric is a plant individual from the ginger family. It has become more standard lately as a cooking specialist in many curry-based culinary dishes, as indicated by nutritionists and Nervous system specialists. Deductively, contemplates have noticed this adaptable zest for medical advantages from the decrease of joint pain aggravation to therapy for an intestinal miracle. However, turmeric is likewise been adulated for emphatically influencing atoms in the mind that help psychological capacity."

18. Chickpeas

Chickpeas have a wide assortment of supplements that are advantageous for brain wellbeing, as per plant researchers and nutritionists."First, they are comprised of complex carbs, which are the essential fuel hotspot for the mind. They likewise contain magnesium, which loosens up veins and sends more blood to the mind. More blood in the brain assists it with working at its fullest limit. I love eating chickpeas in grain bowls or veggie burgers or I concoct some chickpea-based pasta for a straightforward weeknight supper. This pasta has more fiber and protein than customary pasta.

19. Vitamin C Rich Food varieties

Vitamin C-rich food varieties like squeezed orange and strawberries can help support brain wellbeing since keeping up solid vitamin C levels can have a defensive impact against psychological decrease and Alzheimer's infection, according to specialists.

20 Coffee and caffeinated Tea

Caffeine can support your memory, readiness, and intellectual capacity, and has been appeared to help improve test scores and increase your capacity to focus during errands; Espresso and teas can really make you more astute!"

21 The Mediterranean Eating routine

All in all, the best food sources for brain wellbeing for the most part fall into the classification of the Mediterranean Eating routine—an eating regimen that has really been demonstrated to be the best eating regimen for weight reduction. .The Mediterranean eating routine is an incredible eating regimen to follow for the brain since it is calming and has been demonstrated to advance life span and decrease the danger of illness, which incorporates Alzheimer's.

The consequences of an examination as of late show that after a Mediterranean eating routine, it can effectively affect the soundness of our brain, particularly as we age, "The Mediterranean eating regimen is a term commonly utilized about slims down that contain a bigger measure of organic products, vegetables, olive oil, beans, and cereal grains (like rice and wheat). Then again, such eating regimens contain moderate measures of fish, dairy items, and wine and restricted measures of poultry and red meat. The subjects who followed this eating routine were concentrated over the long haul and the individuals who followed it less intently were appeared to have a higher loss of mind volume. Brain volume misfortune can influence learning and memory, particularly as we get older. Yet, the parts of the Mediterranean eating routine appeared to have defensive advantages for the brain.

CHAPTER SEVEN

THE PLACE OF EXTRACURRICULAR-EXERCICES, GAMES

Exercise can help your memory and thinking abilities

Moderate-power exercise can help improve your reasoning and memory in only a half year.

You presumably definitely realize that exercising is important to save muscle strength, keep your heart solid, keep up sound body weight, and fight off constant illnesses like diabetes. Be that as it may, exercise can likewise help support your reasoning abilities. There's a great deal of science behind this,

Exercise supports your memory and thinking abilities both straightforwardly and in a roundabout way. It acts straightforwardly on the body by invigorating physiological changes like decreases in insulin opposition and irritation, alongside empowering the creation of development factors — synthetic compounds that influence the development of fresh blood vessels in the brain and surprisingly the wealth, endurance, and by and large wellbeing of new synapses.

It additionally acts straightforwardly on the actual mind. Numerous investigations have proposed that the pieces of the brain that control thinking and memory are bigger in volume in individuals who exercises than in individuals who do not. Significantly more energizing is the tracking down that taking part in a program of standard exercise of moderate force more than a half year or a year is related with an expansion in the volume of chose mind areas.

Exercise can likewise support memory and thinking by implication by improving the state of mind and rest and by diminishing pressure and tension.

Is it accurate to say that one is practiced better compared to another as far as brain wellbeing We do not have a clue about the response to this inquiry because practically the entirety of the examination so far has taken a look at strolling. "In any case, almost certainly, different types of oxygen-consuming activity that get your heart siphoning may yield comparable advantages.

An examination distributed as of late tracked down that judo showed the possibility to upgrade intellectual capacity in more established grown-ups, particularly in the domain of chief capacity, which oversees psychological cycles like arranging, working memory, consideration, critical thinking, and verbal thinking. That might be because yoga, military workmanship that includes moderate, centered developments, requires acquiring and retaining new abilities and development designs.

Military Workmanship master suggests building up exercises as a propensity, practically like taking a doctor-prescribed prescription. Furthermore, since a few examinations have shown that it requires around a half year to begin receiving the intellectual rewards of activity, he reminds you to be patient as you search for the main outcomes — and to then keep exercising forever.

Focus on an objective of exercising at a moderate power — like lively strolling — for 150 minutes out of every week. Start with a couple of moments daily, and increase the sum by five or 10 minutes consistently until you arrive at your objective.

CHAPTER EIGHT
CONCLUSION

Intelligent quotient levels of the different individual fluctuate; while some have significant degrees of it others are battling with low levels

In the primary case, undeniable degrees of level of intelligence could come from hereditary variables, ways of life, or nutrition. Now and then it very well may be heavenly. In the subsequent case, the majority of these components could be feeling the loss of a larger piece of having a sound keen remainder relies upon you or the activities you're included in(whether negative or good).

We ought to be sufficiently cognizant to comprehend that our undeniable level or low degrees of level of intelligence and buildups of exercises we're engaged with whether positive or negative might be given to our children deliberately or unwittingly.

While your level of intelligence will likely continue as before for the duration of your life, that does not mean you cannot get more intelligent than you as of now are. All things considered, a level of intelligence can gauge just certain parts of your intellectual limits while totally disregarding others. Try to follow the information given here, and you'll have the option to keep your brain sharp, your memory new, and your center solid.